LEARNING TO USE MAKE-UP – THE BASIC PRIN

Learning to use make-up is an exciting passage in a girl's life. In the end practicing what looks good on you will win out, but you should always remember that make-up is designed to enhance your own natural beauty and not hide it – so use sparingly for the best effect.

Follow these helpful tips to greatly improve your makeup experience.
With every season there will be various flattering trends. On the one hand, there is the natural look with earthy and gold tones, and neutral tones for the eyes and transparent but shiny lips. On the other hand, there is the sexier look with darker tones for the eyes from navy blue to purple, and (don't forget black), and dark sexy lips.

ADVICE: Choose a look that works for you and one that you feel most comfortable with and follow the advice that we give you below as you learn what you like and what works for you.

FOUNDATION

The first step in applying makeup is choosing the perfect foundation. This is done by matching the makeup with your skin tone and complexion. Your skin tone will either suit a yellow base, a pink base or a dark base depending on skin colour. Take advice as to which make-up will suit your skin tone best. Always make sure the makeup is well blended and there are no foundation lines around the neck.

Give a touch of something pearlescent to your foundation and you will achieve a modern and flattering look.

ADVICE: Apply your foundation to the entire face. Once it has been applied onto the skin, wait a few minutes for it to absorb, apply a small amount of illuminating powder in the T zone, forehead, cheekbones and chin. Blend it well with a brush for a pearly but natural effect. The result, light satiny skin.

COVER UP & CONCEALER

Brighten your look by using a light cover up which is lighter than your skin tone over your foundation. For any visible blemishes or dark circles under the eyes, a concealer can be used. Just dab it on lightly and blend it in good with the foundation.

ADVICE: Blend it well around your eyes with your fingertip to take away any excess. And that's it, a great look without bags and full of life.

CHEEKBONES & BLUSH

You may want to add a little cheek colour just to make people think you have a natural glow, so give your cheekbones a healthy look with soft rosy natural colours.

ADVICE: Blend blush well with a clean brush and loose powder on your cheekbones. Using a cheek colour brush and this will make blending easier and the result look more natural.

LIPS

Your lips can be brought out by lining them with a pencil, then filling them in with a creamy lipstick. This will give definition and shape to your lips. Glossy lipstick can be used for that stunning look.

If you want a natural look just apply lip gloss on its own – maybe one with a hint of colour in.
On the other hand, if you want to forget the natural look, try a passionate red or a bright pink matte colour. The result, sexy provocative, but natural lips.

ADVICE: Use a well-sharpened lip pencil that is very similar to your lipstick to outline your lips. Do this before applying lipstick so that the colour will last longer and it will be easier to use darker tones. When choosing a lip gloss pick one that protects your lips as well as shines.

EYES

Once your foundation is applied, your eyes are the next important step. Eye makeup is the fun part of applying cosmetics. Use eye shadows that fit your character or to express your mood. You do not want your eye shadow to match the colour of your dress or outfit, but you do want it to compliment it.

Eye Make-up application can take into account your eye shape and this is where practice comes in. Make-up for various shapes is as follows:

Small eyes: Use a light shade of powder for the centre of the lid and a darker shade in the outer edge.

Almond-shaped eyes: Use a light shade of powder from your lashes to the brow, a medium shade on your lid, and a darker shade on the outer third of your eyelid.

Round eyes: Use light coloured shadow over the entire lid and a darker shade in the crease. Apply eyeliner on both the top and bottom lids and use mascara on the upper outer lashes.

Wide-set eyes: Use a darker shade in the inner corner, blending up and out. Concentrate eyeliner and mascara on the inner corner of the eye.

Close-set eyes: Use one colour, varying from a light to darker shade. Start with the lightest shade one-third away from the inner corner of your eye, blending darker shades up and out. Use eyeliner on the outer half of your eye.

Deep-set eyes: Use eyeliner on both the upper and lower lids, remembering to smudge and soften the line.

General Eye Makeup Tips

1. Apply the lightest shade over the entire eyelid.

2.. Apply the medium shade on the lower eyelid.

3. Apply the darkest shade in the outer corner of the eye to create depth.

4. Apply eyeliner with short strokes, starting from the centre of the eye and working towards the corners.

5. Mascara finishes your makeup.

6. Do not wear bold eye makeup and a bold lipstick at the same time – chose either one or the other or the look will be too much. eg. Dramatic eyes and simple lips or Dramatic lips and simple eyes.

7. For a natural look, use browns and neutral tones.

8. For a sexy look, use darker tones, the ones you like the most, from navy blue to bottle green. Or if you like, use grey or black.

MASCARA

Mascara adds the finishing touch to your eyes. For dark eyes, black or dark brown is recommended. Hold the brush vertically to stroke your lower lashes. Then, for your upper lashes, wiggle the brush back and forth at the base, and then sweep the brush upward.

NOTE: Everyone notices mascara so curl your eyelashes beforehand and use two cotes to give them volume.

CAUTION

Just one tip: Do not use any of your friend's makeup (especially eye makeup). Bacteria may be in the makeup because it has been opened and used. This can cause an eye infection and always use only your own lipstick.

USING FACE CHARTS

When you have practiced a make-up look and like the results you should fill in the face chart so that you can reproduce the look again when you want to. You need to fill in all the products you used, noting shades, colours, makes etc. Write down what techniques you used in applying them, what area's you contoured, shaded etc. With eye's which strategy did you choose and how did you blend and the same with lips

FINAL NOTE

Be creative, have fun, enjoy the process and always remember – LESS IS MORE!!

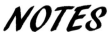

Name of Look _____

Evening ◯

Daytime ◯

Face

Moisturizer

Concealer

Foundation

Highlight/Blush

Eyes

Brows

Eyelid

Liner

Crease

Mascara

Lips

Liner

Lip Color

Gloss

Notes

NOTES

Name of Look _____

Evening ◯

Daytime ◯

Face

Moisturizer

Concealer

Foundation

Highlight/Blush

Eyes

Brows

Eyelid

Liner

Crease

Mascara

Lips

Liner

Lip Color

Gloss

Notes

Name of Look _____

Evening ◯

Daytime ◯

Face

Moisturizer

Concealer

Foundation

Highlight/Blush

Eyes

Brows

Eyelid

Liner

Crease

Mascara

Lips

Liner

Lip Color

Gloss

Notes

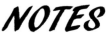

Name of Look _____

Evening ○
Daytime ○

Face

Moisturizer

_____

Concealer

_____

Foundation

_____

Highlight/Blush

_____

Eyes

Brows

_____

Eyelid

_____

Liner

_____

Crease

_____

Mascara

Lips

Liner

_____

Lip Color

_____

Gloss

_____

Notes

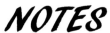

Name of Look _____

Evening ○

Daytime ○

Face

Moisturizer

Concealer

Foundation

Highlight/Blush

Eyes

Brows

Eyelid

Liner

Crease

Mascara

Lips

Liner

Lip Color

Gloss

Notes

Name of Look _____

Evening ⬭

Daytime ⬭

Face

Moisturizer

_____

Concealer

_____

Foundation

_____

Highlight/Blush

_____

Eyes

Brows

_____

Eyelid

_____

Liner

_____

Crease

_____

Mascara

Lips

Liner

_____

Lip Color

_____

Gloss

Notes

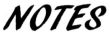

Name of Look _____

Evening ⭘

Daytime ⭘

Face

Moisturizer

Concealer

Foundation

Highlight/Blush

Eyes

Brows

Eyelid

Liner

Crease

Mascara

Lips

Liner

Lip Color

Gloss

Notes

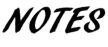

Name of Look _____

Evening ◯

Daytime ◯

Face

Moisturizer

Concealer

Foundation

Highlight/Blush

Eyes

Brows

Eyelid

Liner

Crease

Mascara

Lips

Liner

Lip Color

Gloss

Notes

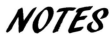

Name of Look _____

Evening ◯

Daytime ◯

Face

Moisturizer

Concealer

Foundation

Highlight/Blush

Eyes

Brows

Eyelid

Liner

Crease

Mascara

Lips

Liner

Lip Color

Gloss

Notes

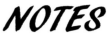

Name of Look _____

Evening ◯

Daytime ◯

Face

Moisturizer

_____

Concealer

_____

Foundation

_____

Highlight/Blush

_____

Eyes

Brows

_____

Eyelid

_____

Liner

_____

Crease

_____

Mascara

_____

Lips

Liner

_____

Lip Color

_____

Gloss

_____

Notes

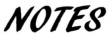

Name of Look _____

Evening ○

Daytime ○

Face

Moisturizer

Concealer

Foundation

Highlight/Blush

Eyes

Brows

Eyelid

Liner

Crease

Mascara

Lips

Liner

Lip Color

Gloss

Notes

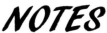

Name of Look _____

Evening ○

Daytime ○

Face

Moisturizer

Concealer

Foundation

Highlight/Blush

Eyes

Brows

Eyelid

Liner

Crease

Mascara

Lips

Liner

Lip Color

Gloss

Notes

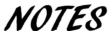

Name of Look _____

Evening ◯

Daytime ◯

Face

Moisturizer

Concealer

Foundation

Highlight/Blush

Eyes

Brows

Eyelid

Liner

Crease

Mascara

Lips

Liner

Lip Color

Gloss

Notes

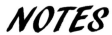

Name of Look _____

Evening ○

Daytime ○

Face

Moisturizer

Concealer

Foundation

Highlight/Blush

Eyes

Brows

Eyelid

Liner

Crease

Mascara

Lips

Liner

Lip Color

Gloss

Notes

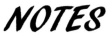

Name of Look _____

Evening ◯

Daytime ◯

Face

Moisturizer

Concealer

Foundation

Highlight/Blush

Eyes

Brows

Eyelid

Liner

Crease

Mascara

Lips

Liner

Lip Color

Gloss

Notes

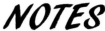

Name of Look _____

Evening ◯

Daytime ◯

Face

Moisturizer

Concealer

Foundation

Highlight/Blush

Eyes

Brows

Eyelid

Liner

Crease

Mascara

Lips

Liner

Lip Color

Gloss

Notes

Name of Look _____

Evening ◯

Daytime ◯

Face

Moisturizer

Concealer

Foundation

Highlight/Blush

Eyes

Brows

Eyelid

Liner

Crease

Mascara

Lips

Liner

Lip Color

Gloss

Notes

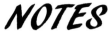

Name of Look _____

Evening ○

Daytime ○

Face

Moisturizer

Concealer

Foundation

Highlight/Blush

Eyes

Brows

Eyelid

Liner

Crease

Mascara

Lips

Liner

Lip Color

Gloss

Notes

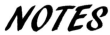
NOTES

Name of Look _____

Evening ⭘

Daytime ⭘

Face

Moisturizer

Concealer

Foundation

Highlight/Blush

Eyes

Brows

Eyelid

Liner

Crease

Mascara

Lips

Liner

Lip Color

Gloss

Notes

Name of Look _____

Evening ⚪

Daytime ⚪

Face

Moisturizer

Concealer

Foundation

Highlight/Blush

Eyes

Brows

Eyelid

Liner

Crease

Mascara

Lips

Liner

Lip Color

Gloss

Notes

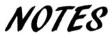
NOTES

Name of Look _____

Evening ◯
Daytime ◯

Face

Moisturizer

Concealer

Foundation

Highlight/Blush

Eyes

Brows

Eyelid

Liner

Crease

Mascara

Lips

Liner

Lip Color

Gloss

Notes

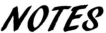

Name of Look _____

Evening ◯

Daytime ◯

Face

Moisturizer

Concealer

Foundation

Highlight/Blush

Eyes

Brows

Eyelid

Liner

Crease

Mascara

Lips

Liner

Lip Color

Gloss

Notes

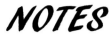

NOTES

Name of Look _____

Evening ◯

Daytime ◯

Face

Moisturizer

Concealer

Foundation

Highlight/Blush

Eyes

Brows

Eyelid

Liner

Crease

Mascara

Lips

Liner

Lip Color

Gloss

Notes

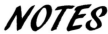

Name of Look _____

Evening ◯

Daytime ◯

Face

Moisturizer

Concealer

Foundation

Highlight/Blush

Eyes

Brows

Eyelid

Liner

Crease

Mascara

Lips

Liner

Lip Color

Gloss

Notes

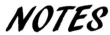

NOTES

Name of Look _____

Evening ◯

Daytime ◯

Face

Moisturizer

Concealer

Foundation

Highlight/Blush

Eyes

Brows

Eyelid

Liner

Crease

Mascara

Lips

Liner

Lip Color

Gloss

Notes

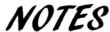

Name of Look _____

Evening ◯

Daytime ◯

Face

Moisturizer

Concealer

Foundation

Highlight/Blush

Eyes

Brows

Eyelid

Liner

Crease

Mascara

Lips

Liner

Lip Color

Gloss

Notes

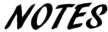
NOTES

Name of Look _____

Evening ◯

Daytime ◯

Face

Moisturizer

Concealer

Foundation

Highlight/Blush

Eyes

Brows

Eyelid

Liner

Crease

Mascara

Lips

Liner

Lip Color

Gloss

Notes

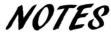

NOTES

Name of Look _____

Evening ○

Daytime ○

Face

Moisturizer

Concealer

Foundation

Highlight/Blush

Eyes

Brows

Eyelid

Liner

Crease

Mascara

Lips

Liner

Lip Color

Gloss

Notes

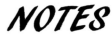

NOTES

Name of Look _____

Evening ○

Daytime ○

Face

Moisturizer

Concealer

Foundation

Highlight/Blush

Eyes

Brows

Eyelid

Liner

Crease

Mascara

Lips

Liner

Lip Color

Gloss

Notes

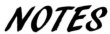
NOTES

Name of Look _____

Evening ◯

Daytime ◯

Face

Moisturizer

Concealer

Foundation

Highlight/Blush

Eyes

Brows

Eyelid

Liner

Crease

Mascara

Lips

Liner

Lip Color

Gloss

Notes

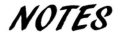

Name of Look _____

Evening ◯

Daytime ◯

Face

Moisturizer

Concealer

Foundation

Highlight/Blush

Eyes

Brows

Eyelid

Liner

Crease

Mascara

Lips

Liner

Lip Color

Gloss

Notes

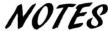

Name of Look _____

Evening ○

Daytime ○

Face

Moisturizer

Concealer

Foundation

Highlight/Blush

Eyes

Brows

Eyelid

Liner

Crease

Mascara

Lips

Liner

Lip Color

Gloss

Notes

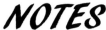

Name of Look _____

Evening ○

Daytime ○

Face

Moisturizer

Concealer

Foundation

Highlight/Blush

Eyes

Brows

Eyelid

Liner

Crease

Mascara

Lips

Liner

Lip Color

Gloss

Notes

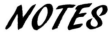

Name of Look _____

Evening ⭕
Daytime ⭕

Face

Moisturizer

Concealer

Foundation

Highlight/Blush

Eyes

Brows

Eyelid

Liner

Crease

Mascara

Lips

Liner

Lip Color

Gloss

Notes

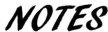

Name of Look _____

Evening ⭘

Daytime ⭘

Face

Moisturizer

Concealer

Foundation

Highlight/Blush

Eyes

Brows

Eyelid

Liner

Crease

Mascara

Lips

Liner

Lip Color

Gloss

Notes

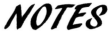
NOTES

Name of Look _____

Evening ◯

Daytime ◯

Face

Moisturizer

Concealer

Foundation

Highlight/Blush

Eyes

Brows

Eyelid

Liner

Crease

Mascara

Lips

Liner

Lip Color

Gloss

Notes

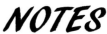

Name of Look _____

Evening ◯

Daytime ◯

Face

Moisturizer

Concealer

Foundation

Highlight/Blush

Eyes

Brows

Eyelid

Liner

Crease

Mascara

Lips

Liner

Lip Color

Gloss

Notes

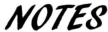

Name of Look _____

Evening ◯

Daytime ◯

Face

Moisturizer

Concealer

Foundation

Highlight/Blush

Eyes

Brows

Eyelid

Liner

Crease

Mascara

Lips

Liner

Lip Color

Gloss

Notes

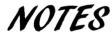

Name of Look _____

Evening ○

Daytime ○

Face

Moisturizer

Concealer

Foundation

Highlight/Blush

Eyes

Brows

Eyelid

Liner

Crease

Mascara

Lips

Liner

Lip Color

Gloss

Notes

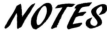

Name of Look _____

Evening ◯

Daytime ◯

Face

Moisturizer

Concealer

Foundation

Highlight/Blush

Eyes

Brows

Eyelid

Liner

Crease

Mascara

Lips

Liner

Lip Color

Gloss

Notes

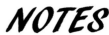

Name of Look _____

Evening ⊙

Daytime ⊙

Face

Moisturizer

Concealer

Foundation

Highlight/Blush

Eyes

Brows

Eyelid

Liner

Crease

Mascara

Lips

Liner

Lip Color

Gloss

Notes

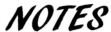

Name of Look _____

Evening ◯

Daytime ◯

Face

Moisturizer

Concealer

Foundation

Highlight/Blush

Eyes

Brows

Eyelid

Liner

Crease

Mascara

Lips

Liner

Lip Color

Gloss

Notes

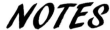

Name of Look _____

Evening ◯
Daytime ◯

Face
Moisturizer

Concealer

Foundation

Highlight/Blush

Eyes
Brows

Eyelid

Liner

Crease

Mascara

Lips
Liner

Lip Color

Gloss

Notes

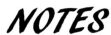

Name of Look _____

Evening ◯

Daytime ◯

Face

Moisturizer

Concealer

Foundation

Highlight/Blush

Eyes

Brows

Eyelid

Liner

Crease

Mascara

Lips

Liner

Lip Color

Gloss

Notes

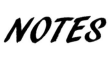

NOTES

Name of Look _____

Evening ◯

Daytime ◯

Face

Moisturizer

Concealer

Foundation

Highlight/Blush

Eyes

Brows

Eyelid

Liner

Crease

Mascara

Lips

Liner

Lip Color

Gloss

Notes

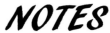

Name of Look _____

Evening ⭕

Daytime ⭕

Face

Moisturizer

Concealer

Foundation

Highlight/Blush

Eyes

Brows

Eyelid

Liner

Crease

Mascara

Lips

Liner

Lip Color

Gloss

Notes

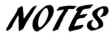

NOTES

Name of Look _____

Evening ◯

Daytime ◯

Face

Moisturizer

Concealer

Foundation

Highlight/Blush

Eyes

Brows

Eyelid

Liner

Crease

Mascara

Lips

Liner

Lip Color

Gloss

Notes

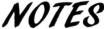